By the same author:

WHY GROW OLD?
and
THE A TO Z OF GOOD HEALTH

THREE WAYS TO TOTAL HEALTH

Vernon Lloyd-Jones
L.C.S.P. (Phys.)

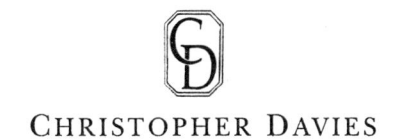

CHRISTOPHER DAVIES

FIRST IMPRESSION 1993

Copyright © Vernon Lloyd-Jones

Published by
Christopher Davies (Publishers) Ltd.
P.O. Box 403, Sketty
Swansea, SA2 9BE

*All rights reserved. No part of this publication may
be reproduced, stored in a retrieval system,
or transmitted, in any form or by any means,
electronic, mechanical, photocopying, recording
or otherwise, without the prior permission of
Christopher Davies (Publishers) Ltd.*

ISBN 0 7154 0726 0

*Printed in Wales by
Dinefwr Press
Rawlings Road, Llandybïe
Dyfed, SA18 3YD*

CONTENTS

Foreword	7
Introduction	9
Ginseng	11
Ginseng Availability	12
How Does Ginseng Work?	13
Ginseng Therapy	14
Ginseng and the Ageing Process	15
Is Ginseng an Aphrodisiac?	16
Further Observations on Ginseng	16
Conclusion	17
Evening Primrose Oil	19
Essential Fatty Acids	20
Evening Primrose Oil & Pre-Menstrual Problems	21
Skin Problems	23
Arthritis	25
The Hyperactive Child	27
Multiple Sclerosis	29
Exercise and M.S.	31
Conclusion	32
Royal Jelly	34
Arthritis	36
Skin Problems	36
Women's Problems	37
Stress	39
Conclusion	43
Forward, Forward	44

*Dedicated to all my staff
– without whose help I would not have
had time to write this book*

FOREWORD

As readers of my previous books are already aware, I owe my life to natural remedies. Indeed, twenty-nine years ago the medical profession gave me just two weeks to live, but, thanks to the dedication and skill of a Russian herbalist, I have, for the past twenty-five years been able to continue the practice of natural medicine.

During those twenty-five years I have been totally involved in the field of alternative medicine – with particular experience of the distribution of the products available. Therefore I have watched the growth of the natural health movement from its very early days. In those early days, anybody who acclaimed the virtues of health foods and natural remedies was regarded as some kind of freak. Indeed the first wholefood restaurant that opened in London gloried under the name of 'Cranks'! Today, as you all know, the health food movement is now internationally accepted as the normal way of life, and we now question the safety of food additives and processing. What a transformation over those twenty-five years! I like to think that I may have played some small part in this development – by virtue of ten years of regular radio broadcasts, hundreds of lectures and discussions with local organisations, and twenty-five years of retail distribution. Because of this experience I am constantly asked questions by customers, listeners and patients about the availability, uses and values of the increasing number of preparations in the news. Recently the ever-recurring questions concern three particular products, namely *Ginseng, Evening Primrose Oil* and *Royal Jelly.*

In my opinion these three are the most valuable natural remedies available to us today, but, because of their very popularity, it is evident that there are many misconceptions about their use. Much of this confusion has been brought about by the popular press, ever anxious to increase its circulation by a dramatic (although often misleading) headline, leading to consequent ill-informed gossip in kitchens, clubs and bars. Therefore, it is my intention in this book to clarify the background, current thinking and uses of this amazing trio of nature's products.

INTRODUCTION

Nearly everything we eat is derived from the plant world or from the animals that live on plants, but it is also true that many of our natural foods can also be used as medicines. Liquorice, honey and garlic, were all widely used in previous centuries. In contrast, over the last half century, Western medical practitioners have tended to ignore these natural remedies, placing their faith in the much hyped chemical products of the modern pharmaceutical industry. Our conventional doctors have suggested that those natural remedies were alright for our antique country cousins, but not good enough for their sophisticated scientific use.

Over the last few years, however, there has been an increasing awareness of the long term side effects of many modern drugs, and the medical profession are once again showing interest in those very same natural remedies which they have hitherto belittled. At this point I feel that it is well worth pointing out that this traditional natural medicine has been developed over thousands of years, and, in my view, the vast experience of practical use over thousands of years is worth much much more than the short term documented evidence giving so called scientific proof of the safety and effectiveness of modern drugs. Critics of natural therapy invariably ask for scientific proof, but it is worth noting that the sort of clinical trials that are now demanded cost literally millions of pounds and consequently it is impossible to produce the evidence required, apart for a few widely used products.

Again, one wonders why such credence is placed in this much vaunted clinical evidence, when one considers the awful consequences of *Opren* or *Thalidomide*, and even the *Dalkon Shield* methods of birth control. These are but a few of clinically proven remedies which have produced disastrous results. Small wonder, therefore, that the medical profession are showing renewed interest in natural remedies. With this in mind we will now consider the first of what I believe to be the three most valuable natural remedies available today.

GINSENG

Since ginseng has been used medicinally for literally thousands of years in the Orient, particularly in China, it is not surprising that many books have been written about it. For my part I do not propose to write at length about the technicalities of ginseng, but merely to make my own observations about the benefits claimed by regular users of ginseng, together with a few comments on the 'mystique' surrounding it.

Ginseng has always been known as *Panax* ginseng – this word *panax* meaning 'all healing', which in itself surely describes the properties of ginseng. Since this description of ginseng as all healing has survived for tens of centuries, this alone must prove the enormous faith in its medicinal properties.

Basically Korean ginseng is a deciduous plant which is normally cultivated for six or seven years before the root is harvested for its medicinal properties. This root is often referred to as the 'Man Root', because it is reputed to resemble the shape of a man, if one has a good imagination! In Korea ginseng is still cultivated in the traditional manner; prayers are said before the seeds are sown. After the nutritious root has been harvested some six or seven years later, nothing else will grow in that soil for a further six years, all the vital ingredients having been used by the ginseng. The Chinese still regard ginseng as their most important medicine – indeed one of their old hymns describes it as 'The Earth Root which strengthens the nerves'. An eighteenth century Emperor is even reputed to have waged war over possession of the best ginseng growing areas! Whilst they may not wage war over ginseng today, there are still some hospitals in China where they use it before and after clinical operations in the firm belief that the patient's overall resistance and immune system will be greatly improved. Thus the patient is considered to be more likely to have successful surgery with a speedier recovery, than if modern drugs were used. With such credence in the power of ginseng in the Far East, then it behoves us in the so-called sophisticated West to seriously think about its wider general use in medical therapy.

Ginseng Availability

There are two main types of ginseng generally available today, namely Korean ginseng and Siberian ginseng. Korean ginseng is the traditional form, and is considered by some people to be a little more potent than its Russian cousin! Strictly speaking it can be argued that Siberian ginseng is not a true ginseng, its correct name being 'Eleutherococcus Senticosus', but to all intents and purposes, and certainly as far as the comments in this book are concerned, we will consider the two forms as having the same clinical properties.

Of course the Chinese have traditionally taken ginseng in its original root form, but in the West the most popular presentation is in a tablet or capsule, although elixirs are available – as well as the dried root. The Chinese tend to take higher doses than we do – because they are steeped in the tradition of just how effective ginseng is. It has been said that some families take as much as they can afford, which certainly says a lot for the safety of ginseng, as well as for its freedom from side effects! Meanwhile, in Europe there is always a suggested normal dose on the packaging, which can, of course, be varied according to the need of the user.

With the ever-increasing popularity of ginseng, it is inevitable that some of my readers may have come across more esoteric uses for it – indeed I have seen ginseng Shampoo and soap, but I will refrain from passing clinical judgement on these!

How Does Ginseng Work?

If I could answer that question, then I would indeed be unique, because, despite all the research that has gone into its mode of action nobody has yet been able to explain the exact function of ginseng. Many have made numerous suggestions and theories about it but, so far, there has been no proven clinical explanation. Suffice to say that ginseng is generally regarded as an 'Adaptogen' – that is to say that it tends to adapt to the body's needs. For example it was used to treat two groups of dogs, one group with a raised blood sugar level and the other with a lowered blood sugar level. In both groups the blood sugar level was restored to near-normal after the administration of ginseng. Similarly, elderly patients with blood pressure problems have been treated with ginseng: those with high blood pressure reported a lowering of that level, whilst those with low blood pressure reported an increased pressure. In summary, it can be said that ginseng tends to restore impaired body functions to their norm. Little wonder, therefore, that it is so universally applauded, and, at this stage, I will now make a few observations on its use as a medicine.

Ginseng Therapy

While it would be rash to suggest ginseng as a cure for specific illness, it is certainly recommended to improve overall health and to build up resistance to disease. In other words ginseng is a highly effective tonic – a word which is very familiar to the 'over forty-fives'! That is why I encourage the use of ginseng as a form of preventive medicine. This is a concept familiar to people from the Eastern Countries, whereas we, in the West, take action only when we *are* ill! How much better to avoid the illness in the first place.

In today's fast moving world none of us can avoid stress in one form or another, and most of us can cope with reasonable levels of it, but beyond certain limits, stress undoubtedly causes all sorts of health problems, even to the extent of a breakdown of natural immunity. I will explain what I mean by varying levels of stress. For instance, being confronted by every traffic light on red whilst driving to work, is a problem that most of us can handle comfortably. There is the stress of noise: pneumatic drills, ghetto blasters in the street or on the beach, the incessant din on the factory floor. Some of us can cope with these stress factors quite easily, but they present real problems to others. Then, of course there are higher degrees of stress, often of emotional origin: going through a divorce, fear, grief at the loss of a loved one. This is when ginseng can be of great value and I have seen quite dramatic improvement in people suffering with stress problems.

Considerable research has been carried out in Russia on this subject, particularly with factory workers in a noisy atmosphere. In all cases absenteeism was greatly reduced when the employees were treated regularly with ginseng. As a result of these studies, ginseng is now freely available to the workers, as it is to many members of the armed forces in both China and Russia.

In summary, if ginseng can improve resistance to stress, then clearly it improves resistance to stress related illness, and we all know how widespread is the problem of this type of illness.

Ginseng and the Ageing Process

Today we are living in a world, dominated by youthfulness and I find, at every talk that I give, more and more people are trying to stay young. Now while it is arguable whether or not we can increase our life span, it is certainly true that we can ward off many of the health problems which contribute to the body's degeneration. I am referring to such illnesses as heart disease, diabetes, depression and general lethargy. Indeed, as I wrote in my first book *Why Grow Old?*, it is possible to slow down the ageing process by looking after the inner body as well as the outer. So, when you are at pains to fill in, patch and cover up those tell-tale lines and wrinkles, do give an equal amount of consideration to your diet.

This is where ginseng can play a very important role, for if ever a natural supplement were tailor-made to tone up the overall body metabolism, then surely it is ginseng. The health benefits derived from ginseng therapy have a self-perpetuating effect, for if you are not weighed down with physical illnesses, then you feel better in yourself. You are not then prone to depression, and your outward appearance begins to glow with the confidence derived from inner well being!

Is Ginseng an Aphrodisiac?

Much has been said, and written, about ginseng and its effect on the reproductive system, and, of course, many wild claims have been made for it. As far as I can see, ginseng improves the overall body performance – remember its adaptogenic properties – and, if it improves one's performance in bed! In fact quite a few clinical studies have been conducted on this aspect of ginseng, and it has been claimed that mice reached sexual maturity younger, and remained sexually active for longer, when taking ginseng.

Similarly there have been encouraging reports about the advantages of ginseng in overcoming impotence in older people. Such results are compatible with the claims of ginseng as an adaptogen, and, to anyone who wants to maintain a healthy sex life, I would say 'carry on taking the tablets'.

Further Observations on Ginseng

Having read of the fascinating properties of ginseng, you might well ask why there has been comparatively little interest in the Western world, particularly since it has been in use for thousands of years in the East. There are several reasons for this, not the least of which is the language barrier. Most of the documented evidence of the clinical value has been written in Russian, Chinese and other Oriental tongues. We Westerners are notoriously lazy when it comes to studying those languages and, as a result, books, articles and scripts have not been translated for our consumption. Of course with the increasing commercial interchange with these countries, there is now a much wider understanding of the languages, and hence an increasing interest in all the products of the East, including ginseng. Hitherto it has been the case that we in the West, have elected to consider ourselves as leaders and teachers and have not wanted to be the taught! Here again modern commercial interchange is altering that idea.

Another major reason for the apparent lack of interest is the massive power of the pharmaceutical industry and medical training. All their resources have been ploughed into the promotion of modern synthetic drugs, many of which are fast-acting – as well as fast profit producing! Both of these factors have precluded the use of ginseng, because, like all natural remedies, it is gradual in the build up of effectiveness. Likewise there are not huge profits to be made from the sale of ginseng, and the big corporations need high profitability in order to exist.

Conclusion

In summary, I would recommend ginseng as a very effective all round tonic of value to all age groups. Younger folk do not need to take it on a routine basis, but they would find it helpful at particular times, for example during periods of stress or when high physical demands are being made of the body. For the over-thirty-fives I would suggest it is worth taking on a regular basis, because of its anti-aging properties, as well as its power to build up the body's immune system. This will help ward off many debilitating diseases which we might otherwise encounter.

One final category for whom I consider ginseng as a 'must' is the serious sportsman and athlete, since it improves both mental and physical performance. During a radio phone-in programme a few years ago, a caller corrected me about the universal use of ginseng by the Olympic athletes, pointing out that it was the Russian team that had used it. In reply I asked him who brought back most gold medals. It was of course the Russians, benefiting from the best clinical advice as well as training.

EVENING PRIMROSE OIL

There must be very few people in the country today who have not heard of Evening Primrose Oil. It is currently enjoying much favourable publicity in the press as well as on T.V. and radio. Yet, twenty-five years ago, when I was recommending it for the treatment of women's problems, skin conditions and multiple sclerosis, I was one of just a handful of people who were aware of its existence. Historians claim that the evening primrose has been around for many thousands of years, but it was not known in Europe on a wide scale until the early eighteenth century. It is reputed to have migrated here from the Americas via the ballast in cargo ships, which is why it was to be found in many of the dock areas.

Initially the plant was used medicinally by just a few herbalists for a variety of different conditions, and then, in the early part of this century, research was carried out on possible industrial use. At this stage it was discovered that the seeds of the evening primrose plant contained some very interesting oil. One of its ingredients was a previously unknown fatty acid which was subsequently named *Gamma Linolenic Acid* GLA as it is now generally called.

It was in the late 1950s and early 1960s that scientific work was carried out in this country to develop the possible medical use of GLA. Much of this worthwhile research in the 1960s was carried out by a British biochemist, John Williams, to whom a great debt is owed for his perseverance. The early work went into establishing the value of GLA as an essential fatty acid and also its effectiveness in cholesterol control. Subsequent studies have demonstrated the ever-broadening scope of this fascinating wild plant, which is, of course, now being farmed on a large scale.

Essential Fatty Acids

When I talk of fatty acids I must point out that many of the foods we eat may appear to be of great nutritional value, but in fact they are often very limited in their function. So please do not regard essential fatty acids as those fats that are found in abundance in such foods as ice cream, butter and other animal fats. Basically there are two types of essential fatty acids, both of which we need to maintain a healthy body. Unfortunately, with today's modern processing methods, the linoleic acid type cannot always be converted into the essential form of GLA.

Linoleic acid is to be found in some meats, dairy products and human milk, while other type of essential fatty acid (alpha linolenic acid) is found in soya, linseed and green vegetables. You might well say that these foods are readily available, so why the need for evening primrose oil? The answer is that there are a number of 'blockers' which prevent the necessary conversion processes. These blockers include foods high in saturated fat and those rich in cholesterol.

A deficiency in essential fatty acid intake can lead to all sorts of problems, such as loss in energy, skin and hair problems, and even some breakdown in the immune system. These points alone are a key factor when considering the value of evening primrose oil.

Evening Primrose Oil and Pre-Menstrual Problems

According to statistics up to eighty per cent of women readers will understand the importance of this section of the book, and most of you will refer to the problem as P.M.T. This is, of course, the abbreviation for pre-menstrual tension which really is a bit of a misnomer, since more often than not the problem involves much more than straightforward tension. However, for ease of understanding, I will adopt the abbreviation P.M.T. to include all the various symptoms suffered by women during the menstrual cycle.

Among those symptoms which may be experienced during P.M.T. are:

- General irritability and bad temper
- Swelling in hands, legs and ankles, and possibly the abdomen
- Discomfort in the breast
- Headaches
- Tired feeling.

These symptoms usually occur from anything up to two weeks before the beginning of a period, and they certainly explain why many women can feel almost suicidal during this time. Fortunately, P.M.T. is now widely acknowledged as a clinical problem. Until comparatively recently, women were told that it was all in the mind, and the best thing they could do was to learn to live with it. The fact that it is recognised as a problem still doesn't make it any easier for the unfortunate sufferer (or indeed the unfortunate husband and fellow workers) unless positive steps are taken to remedy the situation.

There are a number of factors which are thought to contribute to P.M.T. and among them is that sufferers are low in essential fatty acids. This is why a great deal of research has gone into the treatment of P.M.T. with evening primrose oil. Doctors, both here and in America, have found that the administering of evening primrose oil has brought noticeable symptomatic relief, particularly when supplemented with vitamin B6 and vitamin E. Further benefits were recorded when attention was paid to the diet regime. P.M.T. sufferers should avoid what I call the 'rubbishy' foods. They should cut down on their sugar intake, reduce their consumption of tea and coffee and also salt. Some women also find relief if they supplement their diet with zinc, and relatively high doses of vitamin C. Sufferers can experiment with the specific supplementation, but in all cases I would recommend taking evening primrose oil: in severe cases 1gm three times daily, and, in less severe cases, half this dosage. Following the above guidelines, research has shown that sixty per cent of women have obtained total relief, and a further twenty per cent at least partial relief. In conclusion, I would suggest that evening primrose oil be taken with food.

Skin Problems

Over the years I have treated many people suffering from a number of different skin complaints, both children and adults. As you would expect, eczema often presents itself as a common problem, and here I have seen some amazing results when using evening primrose oil. This applies equally to babies as well as adults and older children. Infantile eczema is quite a common occurrence and it is considered to be hereditary in origin by one school of thought. It is often found that if one of the parents suffers from either eczema or asthma these two illnesses tend to be passed down through the generations. High doses of evening primrose oil can prove very effective: if the baby is unable to swallow the oil from the capsule, then it can be administered by rubbing the oil on the inner fleshy part of the arms and behind the knees. Again diet is of great importance, and often the child will be found to be allergic to dairy products. In such cases the soya alternatives are of great advantage – as well as goat's milk and its derivatives. Other types of eczema which have been treated extremely successfully by the use of evening primrose oil are seborrhoeic eczema, allergic eczema, and pompholyx eczema. Although some babies do suffer from seborrhoeic eczema it is normally encountered in adults. It usually manifests itself on the scalp, where it causes bad dandruff, and sometimes spreads to the face, causing red blotches, dryness and scaling.

Allergic eczema is not uncommon, and the important thing here is to try and discover the root cause. Common causes are allergy to the metals from which jewellry is made, hair dyes, and cosmetics. I have encountered quite a number of patients who handle coins very frequently, and also soap powders. Skin tests can be undertaken to try and isolate the cause; a small amount of the 'suspect' is put on the skin and if a rash appears after a few hours then you know you have found the answer to the problem. Many years ago I personally suffered from pompholyx eczema, and I know just how much a problem this can be. I recall going to see a skin specialist who told me that I would have to learn to live with it, but when I read about the development of evening primrose oil I used it together with a daily intake of high dosage vitamin B and C. I have now learned how to live without eczema! Pompholyx eczema affects the hands and feet where tiny blisters form under the skin. The blisters break and the area becomes very painful. Overheating aggravates the condition, nasty eruptions often occurring in the summer. I would advocate that sufferers should avoid nylon socks, rubber gloves and plastic footwear. Bathing the affected parts in a mild solution of potassium permanganate is also helpful in relieving the itchy feeling.

I would recommend a dose of at least 500mg of evening primrose oil (in the capsule form) three times daily – but twice that dosage for adults is often necessary in severe cases. With children who are too young to swallow a capsule, two methods are available. Either break the capsule and rub the oil in the fleshy parts of the skin (behind the knees and elbows as I have already indicated) or alternatively drops can be taken with the normal feed. In all cases vitamin E should be taken with the evening primrose oil, this being essential to prevent the process of oxidation. Most commercial capsules already contain this essential vitamin E, but it is worth while confirming that this is the case which whichever capsules you are using.

Arthritis

There are many different types of arthritis, but they all fall under two main headings, namely osteoarthritis and rheumatoid arthritis. It is a disease which knows no age barrier, affecting old and young alike. Rheumatoid arthritis is a very painful condition, involving inflammation of the tissue surrounding the joints. This inflammation can occur quite suddenly, affecting a number of joints simultaneously, or it may be a gradual process affecting first one joint and then another. The joints become tender and swollen, stiffen up and often become mis-shapen.

Osteo-arthritis involves the breaking down of joints, and is usually the result of a wear and tear process. It occurs most commonly in the knees and hips, and often starts as a result of a fracture. Osteo-arthritis can be a particularly crippling disease. The usual treatment for arthritis is to give pain killing drugs which – while they may well give temporary relief – only camouflage the problem, and do nothing to halt its progress. It is worth noting that a very high proportion of the population suffers from arthritis to a certain degree, but we are often not aware of it because it is only of a mild nature. On the other hand this disease can be of a very severe nature which completely changes the lifestyle of the sufferer. Arthritis patients can encounter difficulty in walking and in doing even the most mundane jobs, such as the opening of a tin or jar. As I have already said, painkillers are frequently the first form of treatment a doctor will recommend, and thereafter the patient may well be given steroids. These may be beneficial in the short term, but, with prolonged use, they can produce some serious side effects.

To date there is no foolproof remedy for this disease, but there are certainly some important steps one can take to help improve the situation, and there have indeed been some very promising results recorded when using some alternative therapies. In the first place it is important that sufferers from osteo-arthritis should not be overweight, as this alone puts a lot of extra strain on the already-damaged joints. Overweight people are more prone to osteo-arthritis in the fingers and hands – which suggests that obesity is a pre-condition to general arthritis, and that the overload on the hips and knees does not, or itself, cause the condition. Therefore I am convinced that diet and the control of one's weight are the vital parts of successful treatment of this disease. Practical experience has also shown that a diet containing too much citric acid can aggravate the symptoms of arthritis. A few years ago, there was a fashionable slimming diet called the 'Grapefruit Diet', and a number of users of this diet started to complain of the onset of arthritis. Conclusion: avoid the citrus fruits! That is, avoid the citrus fruits if you have a tendency to stiff joints and general 'achiness', you can get your vitamin C in other fruit and vegetables. In addition I would point out that there is considerable evidence to suggest that a reduction in the intake of saturated fats together with a diet including evening primrose oil and fish oil can help to relieve the pain associated with arthritis and also help to reduce the inflammation caused by the disease. It is advisable to avoid red meat and increase the intake of green vegetables, fish, yogurt and wholemeal pasta and brown rice and to use skimmed milk only. You will notice that this is a diet high in its vitamin B content.

I would also recommend a daily calcium supplement which will help prevent attacks of cramp to which arthritis patients are sometimes prone. Again, selenium has frequently been taken with appreciable benefit – but for this to be effective, it must be taken in conjunction with vitamins A, C and E. In summary, in addition to a diet low in saturated fats, I would suggest the following supplements:

> Evening Primrose Oil/500mg capsule/daily
> Calcium/250mg capsule/daily
> Selenium/50iu capsule/daily
> Vitamin C/1gm capsule/daily
> Vitamin D/200iu capsule/daily

The Hyperactive Child

Most of you will have probably heard about hyperactive children, but few of you will have encountered it as a personal problem. However it is a problem which affects between thirty to thirty-five thousand families in the country today. When I talk of a hyperactive child I do not mean a naughty boisterous kiddy. There is an abundance of such children, and it is natural that it should be so! No, I mean the really over-active child who just never stays still for more than two seconds at a time, a child who is always repeating question after question, and who is dashing hither and thither, both mentally and physically all the time. This child presents a major problem for the parents and they often find that they themselves are unable to cope with the situation. It can even lead to a breakdown of the marriage. Little wonder that much time has been spent on research as to the cause of such hyperactivity.

Maurice Hansen wrote in his excellent best seller *E for Additives* of the many complex problems associated with hyperactivity in children. He draws attention to the effects of diet and the difficulties caused by food additives. Unquestionably there can be a very positive improvement if a strict diet regime can be planned and then followed equally firmly. The basis of any such diet involves cutting out all food and drink which contain synthetic colours or flavours. In addition to this you then need to work out, by a process of elimination, which other groups of foods are aggravating the hyperactivity.

Some hyperactive children are reacting to environmental problems which may well include over-emotional parents, and quite often the child may come from a family where there is a history of eczema or asthma. Yet again it is frequently found that the mother suffers from P.M.T. or may have endured postnatal depression or even migraine. In all cases I would recommend that the child be given evening primrose oil. Not that this is the be-all and end-all of the problem, but there is considerable evidence to show that a large number of patients will improve, especially when it is given as part of a controlled diet. In those cases where there is the associated family medical problem to which I have referred in the previous paragraph, then I would strongly recommend that the troubled parent should also take evening primrose oil.

Multiple Sclerosis

Multiple sclerosis (M.S.) is a disease of the nervous system which can give rise to some very unpleasant physical effects since it attacks the muscles throughout the whole body. Consequently the patient may suffer with speech problems or defective vision and sometimes loss of balance. The symptoms which first occur are usually a feeling of pins and needles coupled with dizziness and general lassitude. These symptoms can be associated with other causes, so it is vital that a very thorough series of investigations should be undertaken before pronouncing that a patient is suffering from M.S.

I have given several talks to local M.S. groups (I use the word 'talk' because it is a less formal affair than a lecture) and these have given rise to discussions of the different theories as to the causes of the illness. Some say that it is brought about by a virus, whilst others suggest that it the result of a faulty immune system. Whatever the causes of M.S. one fact is clear, the disease is most prevalent in areas where there is a high intake of dairy produce.

Research has shown that there is an unusually high concentration of fatty acids present in M.S. sufferers, combined with a low intake of polyunsaturated fats. Other researchers have indicated that the illness usually occurs in the twenty to forty-five year age group; leading one to question whether stress could be a contributory factor? Certainly I have often found that M.S. patients do suffer from stress. Bearing in mind the nature of the problem with which they have to contend, this is not surprising. With these patients it is important to adopt a very positive attitude and to give them hope for the future. It is in order to inspire such hope that I have written this particular chapter. I am not saying that you can cure multiple sclerosis, but I am saying that it is possible to control it with the aid of special diet regimes and specific supplements.

My first suggestion is that the M.S. patient should follow a gluten-free diet. That is to say he or she should avoid foods containing wheat or oats, and normal white flour. Such dietary control certainly helps the condition a great deal. Secondly I would recommend that the patient avoid foods which are rich in animal fat content, and thirdly it is advisable to avoid foods containing white sugar. Generally I would take it as a rule of thumb to eat things which are 'wholesomely brown' as opposed to foods which are 'refined white'. Do not expect immediate results as a consequence of changing to this diet, but there will be a gradual improvement over the months, and the sustained effort will be well worthwhile. Meanwhile you can eat plenty of vegetables, including potatoes, nuts and sunflower seeds, and drink either goats' milk or skimmed milk, and some of the herbal teas. Chamomile is a good one.

Remember, when you are on a gluten-free diet, it is important for you to take vitamin and mineral supplements to correct any potential deficiencies. As well as going a long way to correcting any deficiency of polyunsaturated fatty acids, research has shown that a high intake of evening primrose oil improves other body defects caused by M.S. Therefore, I would recommend that you persevere with the following supplements in addition to the diet which I have already outlined:

> Evening primrose oil/2 500mg capsules/3 times daily (with food)
> Vitamin C 1gm/1gm capsule/daily

Evening Primrose Oil

Vitamin E 400mg capsule/daily
Vitamin B complex 2 capsules/daily (with food)
Calcium and Magnesium 1 capsule/daily
Desiccated liver 6-10 tablets/daily

I cannot emphasise enough that it is essential for you to preserve with this regime. Have patience and the resultant improvement will be its own reward.

Exercise and M.S.

I believe that exercise is of tremendous importance for everyone's well-being, but for M.S. patients it is a *must* for a number of reasons. Firstly it helps control the oxygen supply (which is vital) and secondly it strengthens the muscles and eases stress.

It is beyond the scope of this book to detail the exercise regime, but there are a number of publications which will give the necessary guidance. Suffice to say that, with any exercise programme, you should always begin with a gentle 'warm up' before going through the complete plan. For those of you who think you could never cope with exercises, I would point out that there are recommended programmes for whatever your particular needs are. Most of them allow for you to be in a sitting position. In particular I would recommend that you pay close attention to the breathing exercises.

General Note
Anyone who suffers from M.S. should neither smoke nor drink alcohol, for very good reasons. In the first place smoking restricts the supply of oxygen to the lungs, and

a good oxygen supply is essential for M.S. sufferers. In the second place, it is worth noting that alcohol is a poison, and it makes no difference whether one drinks beer, wine, or spirits, the ultimate effect is the same. Yes, I know that one may experience a pleasant feeling of well-being, but the overall effect is not that of a stimulant, rather the reverse, resulting in a 'toning down' of the body. In the long term alcohol can cause liver damage which is bad enough for a healthy being, but for the M.S. patient it is particularly serious. Be advised, do try and avoid the two hazardous problems of smoking and drinking, but, if you cannot cut them out completely, do cut them down as much as possible.

Conclusion

In this section I have covered various illnesses which are greatly helped by taking evening primrose oil, and the sceptics among you may well think that it all sounds too good to be true. For how can one ordinary plant be of such value in the treatment of premenstrual tension, arthritis, asthma and skin problems, M.S. and hyperactivity? The answer to that question is that the evening primrose plant contains a high percentage of essential fatty acids, particularly gamma linolenic acid. A deficiency of which leads to many different illnesses. In fact I have only mentioned a few of the diseases where evening primrose oil has proved to be of great value and currently a lot of work is being carried to find it possible use in the treatment of diabetes, obesity, some forms of cancer and heart disease. Indeed I am convinced that evening primrose oil has a big part to play in all our lives – not merely as a treatment for specific illnesses, but also as a preventive medicine.

With that in mind, I recall an incident which occurred some fifteen years ago. One evening I went to a restaurant for a meal, having just recorded a radio broadcast on evening primrose oil. A young doctor approached me and said that he had heard the programme and thought that it was 'a load of rubbish'! I wonder what that same doctor thinks today, after the years of worthwhile research that has gone into it and considering the many thousands of people who have benefited from it! Yes indeed the evening primrose is truly a miracle plant.

ROYAL JELLY

What is Royal Jelly
As most of you will already be aware, there are three types of bee in any colony – namely the drones, the workers, and the queen. Predictably the workers are kept constantly busy during their modest lifespan of some six to ten weeks. This hardly bears comparison with the lifespan of the queen bee who may well live for up to six years. Her longevity may well be attributed, in part at least, to the different diet which she is fed. For the first two or three days in the colony, newly hatched larva are all fed Royal Jelly, a special secretion of the worker bee, by the ever-industrious workers. Subsequently the larvae which will go on to develop into drones and workers are fed a changing mixture which includes raw honey. Meanwhile the queen bee cell is given a constant diet of pure royal jelly throughout her entire lifespan. Small wonder, therefore, that so much interest is paid to this wonderful natural food: if the queen bee can outlive her workers so dramatically on her royal diet, what can the benefits be for us humans! Many, many, attempts have been made to make a chemical formulation of royal jelly, but all have failed – proving, once again, that nature will always have the last word.

The reason for the scientists' inability to synthesise

royal jelly is the fact that they cannot do a comprehensive analysis of its constituents. So far it has only proved possible to isolate about ninety-five per cent of the ingredients and it is the remaining unidentified part of royal jelly which makes it so special. Undoubtedly, it is this small factor which accounts for the many, many, spectacular results reported by patients when using royal jelly. Those same patients when treated with the ninety-five per cent recognised constituents of royal jelly, did not record the same degree of spectacular success.

For the record, chemical analysis has shown royal jelly to contain a comprehensive selection of the 'B' vitamins (including B2 and B6), vitamin C, folic acid, inositol as well as a selection of trace elements of several minerals. In addition there is also present a very wide range of amino-acids, both essential and non-essential, the former being those which we cannot manufacture within ourselves. This breakdown of the known constituents of royal jelly shows it to be a nearly complete form of natural health supplement and add to this that potent five per cent unknown factor, the potential jelly is unique!

I think that everyone I have spoken to must be aware of how much I value royal jelly. I have taken royal jelly for twenty years on a daily basis and it is the first item that I pack in my case when I go away. I have already mentioned in another chapter how I am always being asked if I take all the supplements and remedies that are in my shop – well, my answer to that is that I take those which I consider essential for good health and royal jelly is among the top three!

Although I have seen thousands of patients from all over the world, I am still amazed every week by new reports coming in regarding the successful use of royal jelly in the treatment of an ever-widening number of conditions. For your consideration I will now outline some of the problems where royal jelly has been found to be particularly effective.

Arthritis

I have already referred to the problems of arthritis in the section of evening primrose oil, where I pointed out that there are two main types, namely rheumatoid and osteo-arthritis. The former is where there is inflammation of the joints, and the latter is usually a breakdown of the joints due to wear and tear. There is considerable evidence to back the use of royal jelly in the treatment of arthritis in all forms, but particularly in rheumatoid arthritis. Many Chinese practitioners use royal jelly on a routine basis for their arthritic patients – and they have the advantage of many years of experience of alternative medicine. Several theories have been advanced as to why royal jelly is so effective in the treatment of arthritis, but the most likely explanation is that royal jelly is an excellent natural source of pantothenic acid, and arthritic sufferers are usually found to be deficient in pantothenic acid. I would, at this point, re-emphasise the advantage of following a vegetarian diet, or – if this is not acceptable – at least follow a diet free of red meat and where the intake of citrus products is minimal.

Skin Problems

Practical experience shows royal jelly can excellently aid the treatment of various skin conditions such as acne, eczema, dermatitis and psoriasis. I put this down to the ingredients to be found in royal jelly which are already recognised as effective treatment, for example vitamin B6, biotin and sulphur. Acne, a problem particularly prevalent with teenagers, is basically inflammation of the hair roots and often manifests itself in the form of blackheads; royal jelly is very effective in both the treatment and prevention of this complaint.

Dermatitis, a localised inflammation of the skin, usually presents itself in the form of a rash, and is often due to some type of allergy; here, again, royal jelly has proved to be beneficial. Psoriasis, similarly, is sometimes attributed to allergy or to circulatory problems and royal jelly has produced truly amazing results. It can be applied externally as well as being taken orally.

A common factor with nearly all skin conditions is that they are aggravated by stress, and this is an additional reason for the success of royal jelly because it is so effective in the treatment of stress. It is worth pointing out here, that it is also very important to watch your diet carefully if you suffer from any skin problem. In essence, try and cut out sugar, salt and coffee and follow a regime rich in green vegetables and fresh fruit (other than citrus), use skimmed or goats' milk.

Women's Problems

When talking of women's problems, I suppose the first thing one tends to think of is pre-menstrual tension (P.M.T.), but I also consider the menopause, morning sickness and post-natal depression often to be really serious complaints. In all cases royal jelly has much to offer the sufferer. *Pre-menstrual tension* is a problem which many women have had to endure over the years, without much sympathy from the medical profession. At long last, however, there seems to be a greater awareness of P.M.T. as a real problem, and it is acknowledged that treatment is often necessary. Yes, that 'bloated' feeling is fairly easy to treat with the help of diuretics, but the depression, irritability and bizarre behaviour patterns are in a different league. Here the benefits of royal jelly come to the fore because of the B vitamin content, particularly vitamin B6. This, in combination with the evening primrose oil, is of great help during the P.M.T. phase.

Depression and irritability can occur during *Menopause*, and for the same reason royal jelly is of great value to the sufferer. It also seems to be effective in treating the attendant 'hot flushes' but I will not attempt to explain why – perhaps alleviation of anxiety controls the flushes?

Morning sickness is a problem with which most women have to cope at some time or other, and although endured in a good cause, it can still be quite distressing. I have had many reports from pregnant women who say that their sickness has been greatly reduced once they are taking royal jelly, and this they have in common with two of the very prominent 'Royals'. They have both taken royal jelly through successive pregnancies, and this certainly implies its safety as well as its effectiveness, for princesses and duchesses are given the very best possible advice!

Post natal depression can be a very severe illness for some new mothers, and it does sometimes last for many months. Depression, coupled with the newly acquired responsibility of looking after a demanding infant, is often very daunting and can lead to totally irrational behaviour in extreme cases. Yet again royal jelly can come to the rescue insofar as it will lift the depression and will enable 'mum' to cope with the extra physical demands now being made on her. It is worth noting that the last two conditions (morning sickness and post-natal depression) can be part and parcel of the *pregnancy*, and although pregnancy itself is not a normal health 'problem', indeed quite the reverse, I would strongly advise any pregnant woman to take royal jelly for the extra nutritional benefits to be gained. It will help both mother and baby, and mum will be more able to cope physically after the birth.

Stress (including Nervous Disorders and Insomnia)

Nervous disorders, usually the results of some form of stress, are one of the major problems of modern society. Recently I did a daily phone-in radio programme during one whole week. The subject was exclusively on stress and the lines were jammed each day. Such is the magnitude of the problem.

Of course there are different levels of stress. For example the day to day problems at work, which we are usually able to deal with or the emotional stress we can suffer when we lose a loved one. In some cases we need help to cope with this. Only this week a young lady came to me for help as a result of a change in lifestyle. She was about to be married, and what with the problems of the wedding preparations coupled with moving house and embarking on a new life, she felt completely overwhelmed and unable to cope with all the pressure. Often I see people who about to take their driving test and the degree of stress that they suffer is very noticeable. Middle-aged women often endure stress when their children leave home and this is often exacerbated by the problems of the menopause. All these are stress problems, but they represent different levels of stress.

A few weeks ago a man brought his wife to me because she was suffering from nervous tension and he told me that he kept telling her to 'snap out of it'. I told him not to say this as it can be very damaging to the patient. It isn't easy to control nervous problems. Indeed, if it were, life would be wonderful. Nerves are a vital part of the body's machinery so never treat their malfunction lightly; never submit them to unnecessary pressure, and always heed any warning signs. I would suggest that you never undergo long periods of intense work without some form of relaxation in between times. Similarly if you become aware of a heightening of nervous pressure, then take evasive action to decrease that pressure: alter your timetable, discuss the problem with an outsider who may be able to give you more objective viewpoint, or even go back to square one and start all over again.

Many of the patients I see are taking some form of tranquilliser or sleeping tablet and although, in my opinion, it may be alright in the short term, I do not believe that anyone can artificially deaden the nerves and get away scot-free over a long period of time. To me, it compares with going under an anaesthetic, quite nice but not so pleasant when you are coming out of it. As a result there are a lot of people who are habitually hooked on tranquillisers, and they are only half living and not enjoying life as they should be. It seems barely credible, but last year I saw a lady from Swansea who was frightened by the local bombing raids during the last world war, and at that time she was prescribed tranquillisers. Fifty years later she is still on tranquillisers which is astounding. The bombing of Swansea ended in 1944 and so should her intake of tranquillisers!

A great many patients I have seen over the years complain of difficulty in sleeping, and most of them have been prescribed some form of drug or other. Yes, they do seem to work quite well at first, but after a time they become less effective and then the vicious circle begins: either you take stronger drugs or you try and live without any. In either event you could end up with depression, in the first case because you can't sleep and in the second because it is a clinical fact that the long term side effect of some tranquillisers is chronic depression. Consequently my advice is to take tranquillising drugs only for a short period and then wean yourself off them very gradually (possibly under medical supervision). The important thing is to alert your doctor to the fact that you have been taking this sort of drug for more than a few weeks. He is invariably very busy and may well have overlooked your case and meanwhile the receptionist issues you repeat prescriptions.

Today, as I write this book, a report has been published by Charles Medawar, an expert on drug safety policy and director of a very reputable research group *Social Audit*, in which he states that ten thousand people in Britain are in hospital as the result of the side effects of drugs. He blames human error for some problems, but also claims that the law encourages secrecy about side effects. Estimates suggest that people suffering wholly or largely from adverse drug reactions occupy between three and five per cent of hospital beds in the U.K. He continues: 'evidence suggests that drug injury is often avoidable, that standards of drug treatment are often poor and that the quality of care is sometimes bad'. The report says that the use of the benzodiazepam-type tranquillisers illustrates what is wrong with the way in which medicines are controlled. More than twelve thousand people are currently claiming compensation through the courts for problems linked to addiction. Withdrawal symptoms range from mild anxiety to confusion, even to convulsions and people blame the drugs for losing their jobs and the breakdown of their relationships. For many years secrecy about side effects meant the risk of addiction, and around twenty million prescriptions a year are still handed out for such drugs. Mr Medawar states that the law makes it illegal for drug companies to release some information which would help patients. The secrecy of which he complains tends to protect the drug more than either the patient or the prescriber. Indeed 'it aids and abets misrepresentation and misunderstanding and creates a lack of accountability – it seems as dangerous as it is pervasive'.

The group which carried out this research has called on the drug industry to give more information to consumers. I can now hear you, the readers, asking how would I treat patients suffering from stress, nervous disorders and sleeplessness. Well, very often I find that these nervous-related illnesses are caused by a variety of nutritional deficiencies, particularly the B vitamins. That is why I always give royal jelly because it is such a rich source of these vitamins. In addition I recommend ginseng together with a diet of raw fruit and vegetables, cottage cheese, brown rice, wholemeal bread and honey. It is also essential for the patient (where practical) to exercise regularly and take daily walks in order to help with relaxation.

Conclusion

I have written at length about some of the common ailments where royal jelly has been highly beneficial, but this has by no means been an exhaustive survey of its full potential. Indeed, I have received many glowing accounts of the effectiveness of royal jelly treatment in such varying conditions as angina, anaemia, asthma, general geriatric problems, M.E. (the yuppie disease) and even persistent headaches.

When you consider that many illnesses are either stress-related or due to a breakdown in the immune system, then this could very well explain why royal jelly is so effective in their treatment.

I make no apology for writing so much in praise of royal jelly, because I have seen so many people's lives dramatically improved through its use. Yes I have heard the comments of a few scientific critics, but their demands for analytical proof are meaningless when you consider the practical results enjoyed by millions of users!

FORWARD, FORWARD

So there you have it – my considered opinion of the three most valuable natural products available to us today. For my part I take ginseng, evening primrose oil and royal jelly on a daily basis, not for specific health problems but rather as a preventive form of medicine and as a means of keeping mentally and physically active. Yes, this amazing trio can certainly keep you 'in good condition' and help you keep up with the fast pace of this modern world. As I wrote in my book *Why Grow Old?*, for the last decade society has been on a youth kick which is unique in the world's history. As a result, although many people say 'age doesn't matter to me', in fact most of them are very much aware of the aging process. Read any newspaper report and age is invariably brought to our attention. Whether it be a famous celebrity or ordinary Joe Public in a local court case, everyone's age is mentioned.

In the course of my work I often give talks to various groups, and afterwards people often say to me that they are 'growing old gracefully'. In effect they are telling me that they are giving in! My advice to everybody is to think positive – you are not growing older, you are gaining worthwhile experience so that your life is benefiting from maturity and giving increased satisfaction. What we all have to come to terms with is the fact that we are living in a young people's world. The proof of this is when you go to any store to buy new clothes, you will find the shops cater for the '18 to 30' brigade. Again many television and radio programmes are geared for the younger element, as are modern eating houses with their fast food offerings and cold drinks in plastic cartons. Well, I for one am not going to miss out on these modern trends and will make whatever effort is necessary to accept and be accepted by current society.

People often tell me that one can't stop the aging process, but it is possible to slow it down drastically. I have – and I know many others who have, with great success. When I quote names of the famous who have broken the age barrier, for example Sophia Loren, Barbara Cartland, Cliff Richard, Gloria Hunniford, Bruce Forsythe, to mention just a few, it is often said, 'well they have plenty of money, it's easy for them'. Let me stress at this point that money has nothing to do with it. More essential is the will to keep with it. Think of people you know who look much younger than their years, indeed some are ageless; walk down any High Street and you will see someone and you think to yourself 'how old?' You just can't tell – that person is ageless. So now you are asking how can I beat this age barrier? Here we go!

Think of your body as you think of a car; our body works very much like a car – a car has a pump, we have a heart, a car has oil filters, we have kidneys, a car uses petrol as fuel, we use food and drink for energy. If you abuse your car it shows, similarly if you abuse your body it also shows.

You can see an old car (identified as old by its number plates) and think 'that's in good condition', and why?

Simply because it has been carefully looked after, both internally and externally. Now we are just the same except we are not compelled to wear number plates to give away our age!

So what I am saying is that diet plays a very important part if you want to look younger and stay healthy. Well-chosen clothes and wise use of cosmetics can enhance the external you (just as good cleaning and polishing make the car look good), but an equally well-chosen diet is essential to keep the organs of the body functioning to the best of their ability.

Now I consider that your diet should be adjusted so that you do not carry too much weight. Remember every pound you are overweight adds a year to your age! Fat is old, while a slim well-proportioned figure is young looking! To help you in your quest to lose those extra pounds, you must be prepared to make sacrifices. You are what you eat, so if you eat less, then there will be less of you! So give up those extra cups of tea and coffee, forego those sweets and chocolates, avoid that cream cake! Don't eat food late at night, because, if you do, then your kidneys have to work overtime whilst you are sleeping. It is like parking your car with the engine running overnight. In both cases you are asking for problems. Another important factor in your effort to beat the age barrier is exercise. It's no good simply looking young if you are not fit. To me a fit person is a person who is full of energy, stamina, and enthusiasm for life; in other words a person who is full of vitality. Now exercise does not have to be of a very strenuous nature to be effective. (I don't want you over-sixties to rush out to play squash and rugby in your search for eternal youth!) In fact, I think two of the best forms of exercise that I know are walking and swimming. Most of you are certainly capable of doing more walking, and if you haven't been swimming for years then start right now! Most of the sports centres cater for swimmers of all ages, and many have instructors for the senior citizen. These instructors are qualified. They have machines to measure your blood pressure and heart beat and they will devise suitable exercise regimes for you.

Now it must be obvious to my readers that the first natural supplements I would recommend to each and everyone of you who is seeking to enjoy a full and healthy life will be ginseng, evening primrose oil and royal jelly. Not only do these three have marvellous preventive properties, but they also help tremendously in the anti-aging process. Other supplements with beneficial properties to complement your health regime would be garlic perles, lecithin capsules (or granules) and S.O.D. (superoxide dismutae). All of these are readily available and have been proved over the years and are equally effective for both men and women.

I can hear some of you saying that this is all very well but you don't want to be taking a fistful of tablets every day, and in any case you will forget when to take them. All right, then you have been catered for – there is now available a single capsule which contains all three of my top trio of natural supplements and you need to take only one daily. It is called *Formula One* and I recommend it as the ideal base for preventive medicine and for keeping young. In addition there is an ever-mounting record of dramatic results using Sovereign *Formula One* in the treatment of such illnesses as arthritis, psoriasis, eczema, asthma, stress and general fatigue, etc. It is in wide use quite simply as an old-fashioned 'tonic' and people taking *Formula One* say that they have more energy and are able to cope with life's daily problems more easily. Most recently I have had reports as to the very effective results in the treatment of the post viral problem of M.E. (the yuppie disease). Indeed this speaks wonders for the value of *Formula One*, because hitherto, M.E. has been an almost impossible illness to treat successfully. So there you have it. If you want to look and feel young and to enjoy life to the full, watch your diet, exercise regularly, and take the important supplements I have mentioned. But last, and not least, THINK POSITIVE!

GOOD LUCK!